FIBROMYALGIA/ CHRONIC FATIGUE

Learn how you can get your life back

Ray D. Strand, M.D.

Printed in the United States of America

First printing 2008

ISDN 978-0-9664075-1-8

Creative: www.tmdesigns-slc.com

PART 1

THE UNDERLYING CAUSE OF FIBROMYALGIA/CHRONIC FATIGUE

My Conversion

I graduated from the University of Colorado Medical School in 1971 and quickly went into a private family practice following my internship at Mercy Hospital in San Diego, California. For the first 23 years of my practice, I did everything possible to keep my patients from taking any kind of nutritional supplements. I told my patients that all supplements did was create expensive urine. I told them that all they needed to do was to eat a healthy diet and they would not need supplements. After all, this is how I was trained in medical school. Even though I really never received very much training in nutrition during my medical school years and absolutely no training in supplementation, I was very strong in my convictions and all my patients knew it.

In the early 1990's, my wife of 10 years at that time was diagnosed with a disease called fibromyalgia. I had been aware of this disease entity for 5 or 6 years; however, it was initially known as psychosomatic rheumatism. Many physicians believed that this was really not a disease—that all of these complaints of pain, fatigue, mental fogginess, and the host of other symptoms were just "in their heads." When my wife was given this diagnosis, I had to do some very serious research. My conclusion was that this was a true disease. After all, I was living with this disease and it was affecting my family and me every day of our lives. The medical community had no explanation or answer for this disease. They merely recommended treating the symptoms with medication and told those patients with fibromyalgia to find a support group and learn to live with it. This was the very course my wife took.

It seemed like year after year my wife just got worse and worse. She had to deal with a tremendous amount of fatigue and body pain. I spent every evening trying to rub out the knots in her shoulders. Eventually, she got to the point that she would have to go to bed during the early evening, leaving me alone with the kids each night.

In 1995, my wife came down with a very serious pneumonia. Even though we were able to clear this pneumonia using IV antibiotics, she was left in a very fatigued state. She was unable to get out of bed except for maybe one or two hours each day. One of my 3 children had to rotate missing school in order to stay home to care for her. This went on month after month, in spite of seeing 4 different medical specialists and being prescribed 9 different medications. When I would talk to my fellow physicians who were caring for her, they could not give me any idea how long it would take for her to recover or any hope that she would ever improve.

It was right at this time that a friend from a small neighboring town came over and dropped off some nutritional supplements that she encouraged my wife to take. She told Liz that these supplements had helped her husband to recover from a pneumonia he had contracted over a year ago. My wife knew very well what my attitude was towards supplements. She came to me and asked if it would be OK for her to take these vitamins. I was truly surprised by my reaction. I said, "Honey, you can take anything you want. Obviously, we are doing everything the medical community has recommended and have gotten absolutely nowhere."

My wife began taking what I learned later to be a high-quality, complete and balanced nutritional supplement along with some additional grape seed extract. To my amazement, my wife began to show signs of improvement within the first week. She was able to be out of bed for longer periods of time, and she was actually able to be more active. Within 3 weeks, she was literally off all of her medication. Within 3 months, she was better than she had been in 10 years. She has continued to improve year after year. Not only has she added 4 to 5 hours to each of her days, she is now able to ride 2 to 3 horses each and every day. As a horse trainer, being able to ride again was the greatest gift anyone could have ever given her.

This entire experience certainly challenged everything I had learned about nutritional supplements. Right before my eyes I had seen the medical community fail to offer my wife any help. At this point, I was not sure if the improvement in my wife's health was the result of a miracle of the Lord or, to my horror, the result of taking vitamins. The next week, I called in my 5 most effected fibromyalgia patients and related my wife's story to them. I told them I had no clue what I just witnessed; however, I would certainly show them what my wife took and give them the opportunity to try the same thing. Every one of them wanted try the same nutritional supplement regimen my wife had taken. None of them had the miraculous improvement my wife had; however, every one of these patients at one time or other within the next 6 months personally had thanked me for allowing them to get his or her life back. All of these patients, including my wife, still had fibromyalgia; however, they were now able to function normally. If they were careful, they each had enough energy to do everything they needed to do. I had certainly developed a new respect and appreciation for the health benefits of taking high-quality, complete and balanced nutritional supplements.

Fibromyalgia/Chronic Fatigue

There are now over 9 million people in the United States alone that have been diagnosed with fibromyalgia or chronic fatigue. Most of the experts in this field believe that fibromyalgia and chronic fatigue are different expressions of the same disease. What is interesting is the fact that 8 out of 9 cases of fibromyalgia/chronic fatigue affect women. The disease can strike at any age, but most of the cases begin in the second or third decade of life. Once a person has developed fibromyalgia or chronic fatigue, most experts believe that the individual will have it the rest of his or her life. In fact, according to Aetna Insurance, 8 to 9 percent of all long-term permanent disabilities are the result of chronic fibromyalgia/chronic fatique.

I find it very interesting that it takes the medical community an average of 8 years to diagnose an individual with fibromyalgia/chronic fatique. I believe this is partly because many physicians wrongly believe that this is just a problem that is just in their patients' heads. To further complicate matters, there is no blood test, CT scan, MRI scan, biopsy, or any other test that will prove that a patient has fibromyalgia/chronic fatigue. The only way to know if a patient has fibromyalgia is for a physician with some knowledge of this disease to do "trigger point" testing. By placing mild, point pressure on 18 predetermined areas of the body, a physician can elicit significant tenderness in the majority of these spots. In fact, the medical literature and clinical trials have established that if 11 or more of the 18 areas tested are positive, then the patient has fibromyalgia. In order to diagnose chronic fatigue a physician must obtain a history of persistent fatigue in their patients for more than 6 months. There are several other symptoms that physicians look for like recurrent swollen glands (especially in the neck area), frequent infections, and low-grade fevers. However, the way most physicians diagnose chronic fatigue/fibromyalgia is by ruling out every other possibility that might be the source of the patient's symptoms.

In the end, this is usually a very frustrating experience for any patient who has developed either of these problems. Many feel the medical establishment is ignoring them or that their physicians do not believe them. Since all the tests a physician runs on these patients turn out to be negative, they continually hear their doctor say that they can't find anything wrong with them. Sooner or later these patients actually begin doubting themselves and possibly avoid seeing a doctor altogether. They are tired of hearing that nothing is wrong with them. Considering the laborious process of diagnosing patients, combined with patients' frustration, it is not difficult to understand why it takes an average of 8 years before patients are truly diagnosed. This is a sad state of affairs and a very poor reflection on the medical community, especially when a diagnosis can be made after a physical exam that includes a careful history and tender point testing. Obviously, the physician needs to rule out any other disease process that could be causing their patient's symptoms. However, once this has been accomplished, he or she should establish the fact that their patients have a true entity called fibromyalgia/chronic fatigue. I must admit that in the past couple of years most physicians are doing a much better job.

Once a patient is diagnosed with fibromyalgia/chronic fatigue, the physician usually places the patient on an anti-depressant, pain medication, muscle relaxant and then tells them to find a support group and learn to live with it. In fact, the FDA has just approved an anti-seizure medication called Lyrica (pregabalin). This seizure medication has been also used for relieve of neurological pain syndromes. The problem is the fact that the patients in the clinical trials only saw a 50% improvement in their pain levels using this drug. Just take a quick look at the potential side effects of this drug listed in Table 1. What is even more discouraging is the fact that many physicians are now prescribing narcotic pain medication, like codeine, hydrocodone, oxycotin (oxycodone), and Duragesic or fentanyl patches (morphine-like drug) for their fibromyalgia patients. Now they not only have a chronic pain syndrome, but are also becoming addicted to the medication we are prescribing.

What are the Symptoms of Fibromyalgia/Chronic Fatigue?

As I mentioned earlier, I believe that these entities are different expressions of the same disease. Therefore, I will discuss the primary symptoms of fibromyalgia first. The hallmark symptoms of fibromyalgia are total body pain, fatigue, and non-restful sleep. Patients wake up as tired as they were when they went to bed. These patients usually complain of pain above and below the waist. However, I have frequently seen them present early in the disease with regional or localized pain. These patients are not only fatigued, but also have a classical presentation that is referred to as a mental fogginess. In other words, they just don't think clearly. They are forgetful and can easily lose a train of thought. My wife talks about "hitting the wall." When this happens, she might as well just go to bed because she is not able to accomplish anything because of this mental fogginess.

The symptoms that a patient with fibromyalgia can present with can certainly be varied and different. It is because of this that many researchers give this disease the label of "the great mimicker." In short, it can mimic a variety of different diseases that a physician

TABLE 1
Potential Side Effects of Lyrica

Lyrica may cause side effects. Tell your doctor if any of these symptoms are severe or do not go away:

- tiredness
- dizziness
- headache
- dry mouth
- nausea
- vomiting
- constipation
- gas
- bloating
- "high" or elevated mood
- speech problems
- difficulty concentrating or paying attention
- confusion
- difficulty remembering or forgetfulness
- anxiety
- lack of coordination
- loss of balance or unsteadiness
- uncontrollable shaking or jerking of a part of the body
- muscle twitching
- weakness
- increased appetite
- weight gain
- swelling of the arms, hands, feet, ankles, or lower legs
- back pain

Some side effects can be serious. If you experience any of these symptoms, call your doctor immediately:

- blurred vision, double vision, or other changes in eyesight
- hives
- rash
- itching
- blisters
- swelling of the eyes face, throat, mouth, lips, gums, tongue, head or neck
- shortness of breath
- wheezing
- muscle pain, tenderness, soreness, or weakness, especially if it comes along with fever
- chest pain

must rule out. The other problem is studies show that people with fibromyalgia also frequently have other serious diseases like rheumatoid arthritis, lupus, Crohn's disease, and a host of other auto-immune diseases. They may initially receive one of these diagnoses only to find out later that they also have fibromyalgia.

Once the diagnosis of fibromyalgia is made, most patients can look back and see how this may have been the primary source of many of their complaints over the past several years. People who have fibromyalgia also suffer frequently with other problems like reflux esophagitis, irritable bowel syndrome (50% of the time), and TMJ or tempromandibular joint pain (again about 50% of the time.) I frequently deal with fibromyalgia patients who were diagnosed with carpal tunnel or tarsal tunnel syndrome and had actually had surgery with no improvement. Apparently, they had EMG's that were abnormal and the doctors diagnosed carpal tunnel as their primary problem. However, these patients generally never saw much improvement because their pain was due to their underlying fibromyalgia.

One of the most frequent diagnoses I find made in patients with fibromyalgia is depression. Cymbalta is an anti-depressive drug that actually has been approved for the treatment of fibromyalgia. Their physician has already placed almost all of the patients with fibromyalgia I consult on some kind of anti-depressant. Even if their personal physician knows they have fibromyalgia, prescribing an anti-depressant along with increasingly potent pain medication is the typical physician treatment for this disease. However, I have personally found that my patients with fibromyalgia do not really respond to the anti-depressant. When I ask if it has helped them they will generally admit, "Not really that much." I feel this happens because patients with fibromyalgia really don't have a true emotional depression. Their problem is what I refer to as an immunological depression. They just don't have enough energy to accomplish the goals they need to accomplish in their everyday lives. This leads to an immunological depression and discouragement. As they improve with the treatment and support I recommend, I hear over and over from my fibromyalgia patients that they are no longer depressed. The anti-depressants really never helped and when they finally begin feeling better they realize they were never really emotionally depressed, but just down because they could not do what they needed to do in their daily lives.

The primary symptoms of chronic fatigue are an overwhelming fatigue; however, they do not have any significant body pain. By definition, any persistent fatigue that lasts over 6 months is considered chronic fatigue. These individuals also have problems with recurrent swollen glands, sore throat, and low-grade fevers. Many of these patients have been labeled chronic mono or chronic Epstein-Barr virus sufferers. However, research has shown that chronic fatigue is a true illness all on its own, and the underlying cause is still really not known. Over 90% of the population will have a positive reaction to the Epstein-Barr virus test and many have had infectious mono diagnosed in their past.

Like I have said earlier, the majority of researchers feel that these diseases are different expressions of the same disease. Even though no one really knows the root cause of these diseases, I personally believe as do several researchers that oxidative stress is the cause. Understanding, at least in part, how oxidative stress can cause this problem will give you some direction in how I am able to have such success in treating this disease.

Oxidative Stress as the Cause of Fibromyalgia/Chronic Fatigue

Even though no one exactly knows the cause of fibromyalgia, there is growing evidence that the root cause is oxidative stress. When I witnessed my wife's nearly miraculous recovery, I started researching work written by Dr. Kenneth Cooper who started the exercise revolution in the early 1970's and actually coined the term "Aerobics." His book was called, The Antioxidant Revolution [Thomas Nelson 1994]. I heard about free radicals and antioxidants in the past, but truthfully, I really did not understand much about the health consequences of them. However, oxidative stress-the dark-side of oxygen-had been linked to over 70 chronic degenerative diseases like heart disease, diabetes, arthritis, macular degeneration, Alzheimer's dementia, Parkinson's Disease, and even possibly cancer. I began to wonder if oxidative stress could also cause fibromyalgia. Unfortunately, little research money was devoted to this disease, and few clinical studies existed.

In his book, Dr. Cooper detailed a problem known as the "Overtraining Syndrome." He had spent extensive time and effort at his Aerobic Center in Dallas, Texas, trying to determine the cause and concluded that it was "oxidative stress." The symptoms of the overtraining syndrome were very much like those of fibromyalgia. In general, those with the overtraining syndrome experience fatigue, muscle weakness, poor stamina when exercising, muscle soreness, frequent infections, and the list goes on and on. Since my wife's similar symptoms improved after taking some high quality, complete and balanced nutritional supplements, what I now call cellular nutrition, I wondered if oxidative stress could explain almost all of the symptoms of fibromyalgia/chronic fatigue. Let's take a look at what oxidative stress really is.

Oxidative Stress

Oxygen is essential for life itself, but it is also inherently dangerous for our existence. As we utilize oxygen within the furnace or battery of the cell, called the mitochondria, to create energy and life itself, we also occasionally create a cellular exhaust called a "free radical." A free radical is an oxygen molecule that has at least one unpaired electron in its outer orbit, which gives it an electrical charge. If it is not readily neutralized by an antioxidant, which has the ability to give it the electron it desires, it can go on to damage the cell wall, vessel wall, proteins, fats, and even the DNA nucleus of the cell. As I mentioned earlier, medical literature shows this process to be the root cause of over 70 chronic degenerative diseases like heart disease, diabetes, cancer, arthritis, macular degeneration, Alzheimer's dementia, and Parkinson's disease. I now believe that this process is also the cause of fibromyalgia/chronic fatigue. We are essentially rusting inside. The same process that turns a cut apple brown or rusts metal is rusting us inside.

It is important to realize that the number of free radicals you and I produce is not steady. You certainly do create some free radicals just in metabolizing your food for energy; however, there are several situations in your daily life that cause an increased production of free radicals. The pollutants in our air, food and water, radiation, sunlight, cigarette smoke, over exercise and medication all increase the number of free radicals we produce. However, one of the greatest causes of increased free radical production is emotional stress.

We are not defenseless against this process. Antioxidants are like giving your car a new coat of paint to protect the metal from rust. Our bodies make a certain amount of antioxidants, and we also get antioxidants from our foods, especially from fruits and vegetables. However, after researching the health benefits of taking nutritional supplements during the past 13 years, I believe that we all should supplement our diet with high quality nutritional supplements to have enough antioxidants to manage the number of free radicals produced. Because of our polluted environment, stressful lifestyles and over-medicated society, this generation is exposed to more free radicals than any previous generation.

Balance is the Key

It is all about balance. You want to have enough antioxidants to manage the number of free radicals you produce. Certainly, it is wise to cut down your exposure to anything that causes increased free radical production by decreasing your stress level, drinking purified water, eating organic foods, and not smoking. However, we are not able to live in a bubble on this planet. The best way to bring oxidative stress back under control is by providing our body with what I refer to as cellular nutrition through nutritional supplementation.

Cellular Nutrition

I define cellular nutrition as providing the body with all of these antioxidants and their supporting nutrients at optimal levels or those levels that medical literature has established as beneficial. These optimal levels have absolutely nothing to do with RDA levels of supplementation. RDA's were developed back in the late 1930's and early 1940's as the minimal amount of supplementation needed to avoid acute deficiency diseases like pellagra, scurvy, and rickets. They have absolutely nothing to do with the levels of nutrients needed to provide a health benefit against chronic degenerative diseases like fibromyalgia.

Concept of Synergy

When you review the medical literature about the health benefits of taking nutritional supplements, the studies will generally just assess one or possibly two nutrients at a time. Researchers will do a study about vitamin E or vitamin C or Calcium or Selenium separately. This is just the way we do our research. We are always trying to find the magic bullet, and we tend to look at these nutrients like they were drugs. However, vitamins E and C are not drugs. They are simply nutrients we get from our foods. Today because of supplementation, we are able to get these nutrients at levels we previously could never obtain from our foods. Vitamin E is a great antioxidant, but it primarily works within the cell wall or membrane. Vitamin C is the best antioxidant in the plasma or fluids of the body. Glutathione is the best intracellular antioxidant. All of these antioxidants need the so-called antioxidant minerals along with the B-cofactors to do their job of neutralizing free radicals.

Vitamin C actually is able to regenerate or replenish vitamin E so that it can be used over and over again. Alpha lipoic acid is another potent antioxidant that is able to regenerate not only vitamin E, but also the intracellular antioxidant glutathione. Therefore, one plus one is not two, but instead, 8, 12, or even 20. These antioxidants work together in different parts of the body against different free radicals. When you also provide these antioxidant minerals and B-cofactors at optimal levels, you give yourself the absolute best chance of bringing oxidative stress back under control. These concepts are critical for the individual who is suffering from fibromyalgia/chronic fatigue.

Fibromyalgia/Chronic Fatigued Patients have Increased Oxidative Stress

My clinical experience with treating fibromyalgia/chronic fatigue in my medical practice for the past 20 years has given me great insight into this horrible, chronic degenerative disease. Understanding the concept of oxidative stress as the root cause of this disease will help you understand why you may have developed this disease in the first place and why cellular nutrition is your best hope of taking back control of your health.

The medical literature shows that there is usually one of three different events that can trigger fibromyalgia/chronic fatigue. The first is a serious illness. The second is a serious injury or trauma to your body (especially to the head and neck area). The third is severe or prolonged emotional stress. Of course, it also could be a combination of any of these events. All three events significantly increase the number of free radicals you produce and can certainly lead to oxidative stress. When the events are severe enough or occur in combination, they can trigger the start of fibromyalgia/chronic fatigue. I have discovered this history in most of my patients who have developed fibromyalgia.

I also have found that certain personality types seem to be more vulnerable to developing fibromyalgia/chronic fatigue. First of all, 8 out of 9 people who develop fibromyalgia are women. I have found that most of these women are often perfectionists who are type A, hard driving, and very successful. Now remember these are broad generalizations; however, it has amazed me how often I have seen this pattern in my women patients who have been diagnosed with fibromyalgia/chronic fatigue. I see some men with this disease, but the overwhelming majority of my patients with fibromyalgia are women who tend to have these strong personalities.

When I first began my medical practice in the early 1970's, I never saw any patients who had fibromyalgia, and I certainly never made the diagnosis of fibromyalgia. I began hearing the term psychosomatic rheumatism in the late 1970's and early 1980's. However, beginning in the mid-1980's I began seeing more and more patients who had fibromyalgia. Today, there are literally millions of individuals who are suffering from this disabling disease. Why is this happening?

It has become apparent to me that because of our stressful lifestyles, polluted environment, and over-medicated society, this generation has to handle more free radicals than any previous generation. One of the best books that I have read on chronic fatigue was written by a Dr. Ali called The Yellow Canary and Chronic Fatigue. Coalminers would place the yellow canary in a small bird cage and then take it down into the mine with them. If methane gas leaked into the mine shaft, the canary would quickly die. Its death served as an early warning sign to get out of the mine as quickly as possible. Dr. Ali believes that women who develop and suffer with fibromyalgia are like the yellow canary. We are all exposed to this toxic, stressful world; however, some of us are more vulnerable and sensitive to this exposure than others. People who develop fibromyalgia are the yellow canaries of this world. In other words, they are just not as able to handle this increased oxidative stress as well as others.

I also look at the change that has occurred with the role of women in our society over the past generation with the advent of two-income families. Being a wife and mother is probably the most difficult role and job in the world. However, because of the financial strain and demand placed on the family today, many women have had to join the workforce. They not only have to fulfill the role as a wife and mother, but also must work a full time job to help meet the financial needs of the family. The sad truth is that most of women who come home from an 8 hour day at work still must feed the family, clean the house, do the laundry, and meet the needs of their children and husband. Society looks on these women as superstars. Remember, that many women who develop fibromyalgia seem to be women who are not only type A, but also perfectionists. They receive most of their self-worth and identity by pleasing others and meeting others needs. These are worthy goals and desires; however, I have seen so many of these individuals eventually crash and burn. The end result for many of them is the development of fibromyalgia/chronic fatigue.

When my mother delivered her children, she told me that she stayed an average of 7 days in the hospital. Back in the 1940's and 1950's this was the standard of care. I did obstetrics in my family practice for over 20 years. I found it very interesting how things had changed. When I would deliver a child, the first question many of my patients would ask me was, "Is it a boy or a girl?" Then the very next thing she would ask was when she could go home, followed quickly by asking me when she could return to work. This all occurred while the patient was still on the delivery table. Expectations have certainly changed.

I certainly believe that the underlying cause of fibromyalgia/chronic fatigue is oxidative stress. This view is also shared by many researchers into fibromyalgia and chronic fatigue (please review the bibliography at the end of this booklet). Understanding it will give you tremendous insight into this disease. It will also allow you to develop an effective strategy in learning how to regain control of your health. Let's take a look at some of my specific health concepts and recommendations when it comes to fibromyalgia/chronic fatigue.

PART 2

GETTING YOUR LIFE BACK

Nutritional Supplementation—Cellular Nutrition

The most important step for fibromyalgia patients to regain their health is an aggressive nutritional supplementation program. I place all of my fibromyalgia patients on what I refer to as cellular nutrition. Cellular nutrition is defined as providing all the essential nutrients to the body at those optimal levels that medical literature has established as beneficial. Within 6 months any nutritional deficiencies should be corrected, and all the nutrients should be brought to optimal levels. This not only creates the synergy that we desire, but it also optimizes your body's natural immune system, antioxidant defense system, and repair system.

Remember, to correct oxidative stress, you must have enough antioxidants available to manage the number of free radicals produced. One of the best ways to begin accomplishing this goal is to try what I have referred to as cellular nutrition by taking high-quality, complete and balanced nutritional supplements. You will not get what I recommend from a one-a-day vitamin. To get the optimal levels, you will usually need to take a total of 3 or 4 antioxidant tablets and 3 or 4 mineral tablets spread throughout the day and taken with your meals. It is critical that your nutritional supplements are manufactured by a company that follows USP guidelines and pharmaceutical-grade Good Manufacturing Practices.

My patients with fibromyalgia/chronic fatigue have much more oxidative stress than the normal person. To bring this oxidative stress under control, my patients need to add what I refer to as "enhancers" to their cellular nutrition.

Enhancers

GRAPE SEED EXTRACT

Enhancers are added to this cellular nutrition to create more effective synergy and allow an even better chance of controlling oxidative stress. The first enhancer I always recommend to my fibromyalgia patients is grape seed extract. This is probably the most potent antioxidant available today. It is 50 times more potent than vitamin E and 20 times more potent than vitamin C when taken with cellular nutrition. If it is just taken by itself, it is only 7 or 8 times more potent than vitamin E and 3 to 4 times more potent than vitamin C. This positive difference is because of the synergistic effect of using grape seed extract with all of these supporting nutrients.

Grape seed extract is not only a great antioxidant, but also it is a great anti-inflammatory and anti-allergen. Most of my patients with fibromyalgia suffer from allergies and too much inflammation in their bodies. Grape seed extract also readily crosses the blood-brain barrier in the brain. This is important because one of the major problems these patients report is what I refer to as a "mental fogginess."

I initially start my patients on 300 mg to even 400 mg of grape seed extract daily. I previously recommended only 100 mg daily; however, I found over time that only about 20 to 25% had a positive response. When my patients started with the higher doses of grape seed extract, I found that nearly 70% of my fibromyalgia patients had a positive response after they had been on this aggressive nutritional support for over 6 months.

COENZYME Q10

Coenzyme Q10 is one of the most important nutrients that is required for the cell to create energy. Since a major aspect of fibromyalgia/chronic fatigue is fatigue, I have found that supplementing with this important nutrient gives my patients a much better chance for a positive response. CoQ10 is also one of the most potent boosters for our immune system. Most of my patients with fibromyalgia/chronic fatigue have a depleted immune system, and I recommend that they supplement their diet with 200 mg of powder form CoQ10 or 60 mg of gel form. The gel form of CoQ10 is absorbed about three to three and one-half times greater than the powder form. Again, it takes a minimum of 6 months to restore the body's natural immune system and to achieve the optimal levels of CoQ10.

CALCIUM/MAGNESIUM/VITAMIN D

Fibromyalgia patients suffer from tight muscle bands throughout their body, but especially in their neck and shoulders. These taut muscles can be partly the result of a magnesium deficiency. By supplementing their diet with additional calcium and magnesium along with higher doses of vitamin D, patients can experience significant improvement. This is why I always recommend that my fibromyalgia/chronic fatigue patients also take an additional 600 to 800 mg of calcium, 500 to 600 mg of magnesium, and 400 IU of vitamin D. This is in addition to the amount they receive with their cellular nutrition.

ESSENTIAL FATTY ACIDS

I always want my patients with fibromyalgia/chronic fatigue to also take either a filtered fish oil capsule or cold-pressed flax seed oil to get the additional essential fatty acids our bodies so desperately need. I prefer the filtered fish oil capsule. These essential fatty acids or omega-3 fatty acids quickly produce our body's own natural anti-inflammatories and can give fibromyalgia/chronic fatigue patients some significant improvements.

What Supplements do I recommend to my Patients?

If you are serious about trying to get your life back, I warn you to not sell yourself to the lowest bidder. You cannot possibly get everything you need by taking a multiple vitamin. Multiple vitamins are based on Recommended Daily Allowance (RDA) levels of supplementation. RDA's were developed in the late 1930's and 1940's as the minimal requirement needed to avoid acute deficiency diseases like pellagra, scurvy, or rickets. This standard has absolutely nothing to do with chronic degenerative diseases or insulin resistance.

Please take time to look at Table 2 (pgs 23-24)

There are companies that are putting almost all of these nutrients into one or two tablets that need to be taken 3 or 4 times daily. I encourage my patients to take an antioxidant tablet and mineral tablet with each meal or at least twice daily. They need to contain as close to the amount of supplementation I recommend in table 2.

TABLE 2		
Basic Nutritional Supplement Recommendations		
ANTIOXIDANTS	The more and varied your antioxidants, the better.	
VITAMIN A	I do not recommend the use of straight vitamin A because of its potential toxicity. I recommend supplementing with a mixture of mixed carotenoids. Carotenoids become vitamin A in the body as the body has need and they have no toxicity problems.	
CAROTENOIDS	It is important to have a nice mixture of carotenoids and not just to take beta-carotene.	
	• Beta-carotene	10,000 to 15,000 IU
	• Lycopene	1 to 3 mg
	• Lutein/Zeaxanthin	1 to 6 mg
	• Alpha carotene	500 mcg to 800 mcg
VITAMIN C	It is important to get a mixture of vitamin C, especially the calcium, potassium, zinc, and magnesium ascorbates, which are much more potent in handling oxidative stress. • 1000 to 2000 mg	
VITAMIN E	It is important to be getting a mixture of vitamin Es. This should always be natural vitamin, and a mixture of natural vitamin is better: d-alpha tocopherol, d-gamma tocopherol, and mixed tocotrienol. • 400 to 800 IU	
BIOFLAVANOID COMPLEX OF ANTIXODANTS	Bioflavanoids offer you a great variety of potent antioxidants. Having a variety of bioflavanoids is a great asset to your supplements. The amounts may vary but should include the majority of the following:	
	• Rutin	• Cruciferous
	• Quercitin	• Bilberry
	• Broccoli	• Grape-Seed Extract
	• Green Tea	• Bromelain
ALPHA-LIPOIC ACID	• 50 to 250 mg	
COQ10	• 20 to 30 mg	
GLUTATHIONE	• 10 to 20 mg • Precursor: N-acetyl-L-cystein50 to 75 mg	
B VITAMINS (COFACTORS)	• Folic Acid	800mcg
	• Vitamin B1 (Thiamin)	20 to 30 mg
	• Vitamin B2 (Riboflavin)	25 to 50 mg
	• Vitamin B3 (Niacin)	30 to 75 mg
	• Vitamin B5 (Pantothenic Acid)	80 to 200 mg
	• Vitamin B6 (Pyridoxine)	25 to 50 mg
	• Vitamin B12 (Cobalamin)	100mcg to 250 mcg
	• Biotin	300mcg to 1,000 mcg

TABLE 2
Basic Nutritional Supplement Recommendations

OTHER IMPORTANT VITAMINS	• Vitamin D3 (Cholecalciferol) • Vitamin K 50 to 100mcg	450 IU to 800 IU
MINERAL COMPLEX	• Calcium	800 to 1,500 mg (depending on your dietary intake of calcium)
	• Magnesium	500 mg to 800 mg
	• Zinc	20 to 30 mg
	• Selenium	200 mcg is ideal
	• Chromium	200 mcg to 300 mcg
	• Copper1 to 3 mg	
	• Manganese	3 to 6 mg
	• Vanadium	30 to 100 mcg
	• Iodine 100 mcg to 200 mcg	
	• Molybdenum	50 mcg to 100 mcg
	• Mixture of Trace Minerals	
ADDITIONAL NUTRIENTS FOR BONE HEALTH	• Silicon 3 mg • Boron 2 to 3 mg	
OTHER IMPORTANT AND ESSENTIAL NUTRIENTS Improved Homocysteine levels and improved brain function	• Choline • Trimethylglycine • Inositol 150 mg to 250 mg	100 to 200 mg 200 to 500 mg
SUPPLEMENTING YOUR DIET		
ESSENTIAL FATS:	• Cold-Pressed Flaxseed oil • Fish Oil Capsules	
FIBER SUPPLEMENT	• Blend of soluble and insoluble fiber	10 to 30 mg depending on your dietary comsumption fiber (ideal is 35 to 50 grams of total fiber daily)

**There are some nutritional companies who are putting together these essential nutrients into one or two different tablets, which need to be taken 2 to 3 times daily in order to achieve this level of supplementation. Look for a high-quality product that comes as close as possible to these recommendations. If the manufacturer follows pharmaceutical GMP and USP guidelines, you will be giving yourself the absolute best protection against oxidative stress.

The essential fats and fiber will give you the added nutrients that are usually missing in the Western diet.

Pharmaceutical-Grade
Good Manufacturing Practices (GMP)

When you are considering which nutritional supplements to take, there are a few important criteria you need to consider before choosing a particular brand of supplement in order to get the quality you need. The nutritional supplement industry is basically an unregulated industry. The FDA considers nutritional supplements in the same category as a food. This means there is no guarantee that what is on the label is actually in the tablet. The FDA is in the process of improving their standards; however, you need to select a company that already manufactures their products as if they were a drug and not a food. The companies that accomplish this goal follow what is known as pharmaceutical-grade Good Manufacturing Practices (GMP). This means they purchase pharmaceutical grade raw products and then produce them with the same quality control that a pharmaceutical company does. Nutritional companies are not required to do this, but a few of the companies are now strictly following these guidelines so they can offer you the assurance that what they have listed on the label is in fact, what is in the tablet.

US Pharmacopoeia (USP)

Your tablets must readily dissolve or it really doesn't matter what is in them. When nutritional companies follow these USP guidelines, it gives you the assurance that at least your tablet is dissolving. Still many nutritional companies do not follow USP guidelines. The government is definitely getting more serious about trying to raise the bar on the quality of nutritional supplements in this country and the FDA is now looking into setting higher standards for the production of nutritional supplements. However, this will take several more years to implement.

A 6-Month Trial is Critical

When I first began working nutritionally with my fibromyalgia/chronic fatigue patients, many would try my recommendations for only a month or two. During the next office visit, they would tell me that they did not note any improvement and that they had quit taking them. I quickly learned that I did not want my patients to even begin with my recommendations unless they were committed to trying them for a minimum of 6 months.

Nutritional medicine is much different than traditional Western medicine which relies on drug therapy. It takes a minimum of 6 months to replenish a nutritional deficiency and restore all the other nutrients to their optimal levels. This is also the length of time needed to optimize the body's natural defense system. Since there is only symptomatic treatment available for fibromyalgia/chronic fatigue in traditional medicine, I felt sorry for my patients who did not give this aggressive nutritional approach adequate time. When they would try this for only a month or two and then quit, they all felt that it just didn't work for them. They needed to try this nutritional approach longer to know if they would be in the 70% category that had experienced a positive response. Now if my patients tell me that they would be willing to try this approach for only a month or two, I tell them not to start at all. They should wait until they are willing to try it for at least 6 months.

Eating a Healthy Diet

Most of my patients with fibromyalgia/chronic fatigue are very sensitive to sugar. It may be because they feel so miserable all the time that when they spike their blood sugar, they at least feel better for a short time. Many of these patients are also not able to exercise normally. Combining decreased activity with a poor diet often causes a weight problem. This is why I encourage all my patients with fibromyalgia/chronic fatigue to eat a healthy diet containing good fats and good proteins and to avoid foods which spike their blood sugar levels.

I have detailed this healthy diet in my book, *Healthy for Life* [Real Life Press 2005], which is available in bookstores or through my website (**www.drraystrand.com**). You may also want to consider joining my Healthy for Life Program located at **www.releasingfat.com**. My fibromyalgia/chronic fatigue patients have increased chance of improvement if they follow my recommended aggressive nutritional supplement program and healthy diet plan.

Exercise is Critical—but Use Caution

While exercise is critical, it is also potentially dangerous for the patient with fibromyalgia/chronic fatigue. Any exercise, especially aerobic exercise, can make fibromyalgia/chronic fatigue symptoms flare. If you overdo your exercise, you may be in bed for the next two weeks. This is why I recommend that my patients exercise only every other day. Start very slowly, and never exercise two days in a row. For some of you this may mean walking for only 5 minutes every other day. After a couple of weeks with no setback, you may try to increase walking for 10 minutes every other day. Some of my patients are able to increase their walking time to 30 minutes every other day, and some eventually are able to work out two days in a row. However, this only occurs over months of gradual increase.

Since exercise can potentially cause a crash, why do I recommend it? I have found that my fibromyalgia/chronic fatigue patients, who exercise carefully, always do better than my patients who do not exercise. If it is done carefully and increased slowly, it is always a very positive aspect to their care.

Weight resistant training, practicing yoga, or stretching seem to be tolerated better than aerobic activity. These forms of exercise can always be slowly added to a very modest and careful aerobic activity, but I still like the aerobic activity to be the basis of an exercise program.

What Can I Expect if I Commit to these Recommendations?

What I have learned over the past 13 years in treating patients with fibromyalgia/chronic fatigue is that improvements come slowly. The average length of time is eight years before a patient with fibromyalgia/chronic fatigue actually receives a diagnosis. In other words, these patients suffer for years before their doctors make this diagnosis. Many of these patients are very frustrated with the medical establishment because they have often been told that nothing is wrong with them and that it is most likely just "in their heads." Even if the diagnosis is made early, they are usually just given a non-steroidal anti-inflammatory, muscle relaxant, along with anti-depressant and told to find a support group and learn to live with it. Let's make no mistake about fibromyalgia/chronic fatigue; it is a very serious and difficult disease. It is a life-long disease, and many of these patients also develop diseases like rheumatoid arthritis, lupus, or some other autoimmune disease. Therefore, it is certainly worth a short 6 to 9 month trial to try to get your life back.

First and foremost, you must NOT discontinue any medication that you are presently taking. You should only decrease or discontinue your medication under your doctor's direction and orders. Obviously, if you begin to have clinical improvements, you will need your medication less and less. However, any changes in medication must be directed by your personal, local physician.

Most of my fibromyalgia/chronic fatigue patients will begin to note some minor improvements during the first couple of months. The most common improvement they report is clearer thinking and less "mental fogginess." Next, they often report an increased energy level. They may also note that their sleep pattern has actually started to improve, and sometimes they tell me that they are dreaming again for the first time in years. The last improvement for my fibromyalgia patients is a decrease in their pain level. Many times it takes at least 6 months for them to note this change.

Initially, many of my patients with fibromyalgia/chronic fatigue rate their energy level somewhere between 40 to 60% of normal. Those patients who improve rate their energy level at 80 to 100%. This improvement seems to continue over several years on the program. In other words, the longer they stay with the program, the better they are year after year.

There is one very important warning. Almost all of my fibromyalgia/chronic fatigue patients who have a positive response to these recommendations will sooner or later have a setback, and their symptoms will worsen again. Remember, their underlying disease is never cured. When this happens, my patients become very concerned, if not outright frightened, because they worry that they will be as ill as they once were. This is a natural fear; however, I usually just recommend that my patients get some additional rest and increase their grape seed extract by one or two additional tablets. They will normally return to the level of previous improvement and again can just take their regular amount of grape seed extract. Some of my patients have actually learned that if they anticipate additional stress or if they suffer an illness or injury, they can increase the dose of grape seed extract to prevent a setback. Then they return to their previous dose when their stress level is back to normal or when they have totally recovered from an illness or injury.

Not everyone improves. However, nearly 70% of my patients will note significant positive improvement if they stay with these recommendations for a minimum of 6 months. One of the main reasons people do not improve is because they do not choose the highest quality nutritional supplement that is available. Since nutritional supplement companies are basically unregulated, it is critical to choose a company that produces a high-quality, complete and balanced product. It is very frustrating for me, since I began practicing nutritional medicine because people will read my books or booklets and then go out and try to find what I am recommending at their local health food store, grocery store, or pharmacy. Then they do not get the responses I have shared with them and they too become very frustrated.

My "Online Medical Practice"— Specializing in Nutritional Medicine

I would strongly encourage you to consider becoming a member of my online medical practice at **www.drraystrand.com**. This will allow you to have direct access to me via an email or phone consult at a very reasonable price. I maintain electronic medical records of my consults and my website is HIPPA compliant (Health Insurance Portability and Accountability Act). You will also have access to my Standard Specific Nutritional Supplement Recommendations for over 100 different diseases including fibromyalgia/chronic fatigue at no additional charge. Whether you choose to receive my Standard Specific Recommendations or want to consult me personally, I believe it is certainly worth the time, money, and effort to give yourself an opportunity to regain your health.

Complete access to this website costs only $49 US annually and not only does it allow you to receive my bi-monthly newsletters and frequent health nuggets, but you also have direct access to all the resources on this website:

- Immediate access to a variety of resources that will educate, motivate, and guide you into those effective healthy lifestyles that will give you the absolute best chance of protecting or regaining your health
- You will receive periodic emails explaining the health benefits of taking high-quality, complete and balanced nutritional supplements
- You will receive my Bi-Monthly Healthy for Life Electronic Newsletter
- You will have access to my standard specific nutritional recommendations for over 100 different diseases many of which have been translated into French and Spanish.
- Members have the privilege to have direct access to me via an email or phone consult at a very reasonable charge. A confidential electronic medical record will be established for each member who consults me directly for better continuity of care.
- Members have the ability to order bloodwork through my online medical practice at a very reasonable charge.

I have been able to help literally thousands of patients with fibromyalgia/chronic fatigue. Most of these patients have lost all hope of getting their health and life back. How valuable is to you to possibly be able to get your life and health back? Check out my website at **www.drraystrand.com** or visit with the individual who shared this booklet with you.

BIBLIOGRAPHY

Arnold, L.M., et al. "A 14-week, Randomized, Double-Blinded, Placebo-Controlled Monotherapy Trial of Pregabalin in Patients with Fibromyalgia." *Journal of Pain.* June (2008)

Bagis, S., et al. "Free Radicals and Antioxidants in Primary Fibromyalgia: An Oxidative Stress Disorder?" *Rheumatology International* 3. (2005): 188-190.

Fulle, S., et al. "Specific Oxidative Alterations in Vastus Lateralis Muscle of Patients with the Diagnosis of Chronic Fatigue Syndrome." *Free Radical Biology and Medicine* 29. (2000): 1252-1259.

Gur, A., Okatayoglu, P., "Central Nervous System Abnormalities in Fibromyalgia and Chronic Fatigue Syndrome: New Concepts in Treatment." *Current Pharmaceutical Design* 14. (2008): 1274-1294.

Lister, R. E., "An Open, Pilot Study to Evaluate the Potential Benefits of Coenzyme Q10 Combined with Ginkgo Biloba Extract in Fibromyalgia Syndrome." *Journal of International Medical Research* 30. (2002): 195-199.

Ozgocmen, S., Ozyurt, H., et al. "Current Concepts in the Pathophysiology of Fibromyalgia: The Potential Role of Oxidative Stress and Nitric Oxide." *Rheumatology International* 7. (2006): 585-597.

Pall, M. L., "Common Etiology of Posttraumatic Stress Disorder, Fibromyalgia, Chronic Fatigue Syndrome and Multiple Chemical Sensitivity via Elevated Nitric Oxide/Peroxynitrite. *Medical Hypotheses* 57. (2006): 139-145.

Wang, H., Moser, M., et al. "Circulating Cytokine Levels Compared to Pain in Patients with Fibromyalgia—A Prospective Longitudinal Study Over 6 Months." *Journal of Rheumatology,* June (2008).

ABOUT THE AUTHOR

Ray D. Strand, M. D., graduated from the University of Colorado Medical School and finished his post-graduate training at Mercy Hospital in San Diego, California. He has been involved in an active private family practice for the past thirty years, and has focused his practice on nutritional medicine over the past ten years while lecturing internationally on the subject. He is also the author of several best-selling books that includes *What Your Doctor Doesn't Know About Nutritional Medicine, Death by Prescription,* and *Releasing Fat.* He has also lectured across the United States, Canada, Australia, and New Zealand on preventive and nutritional medicine. Dr. Strand lives on a horse ranch in South Dakota with his lovely wife, Elizabeth. They have three grown children, Donny, Nick, and Sarah.

Order Dr. Strand's books and check out his web pages at:
www.drraystrand.com
or
www.releasingfat.com

Health Concepts
P. O. Box 9226
Rapid City, SD 57709

ADDITIONAL BOOKS
Written by Dr. Ray Strand

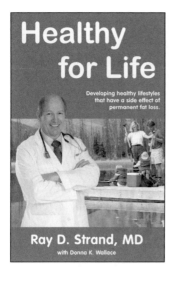

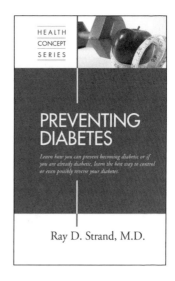

We are in the midst of the diabetes and obesity epidemics. Dr. Strand details the underlying cause for over 90% of the cases of diabetes and obesity—insulin resistance. Learn how you can prevent becoming diabetic as you establish your healthy weight by firmly establishing healthy lifestyles that improve insulin sensitivity.

Our lifestyles are the major determining factor in what kind of disease or diseases we will end up developing. This is even truer when it comes to diabetes whether or not you are genetically predisposed to this disease. Dr. Strand details the problem with the modern day epidemic of diabetes and it consequences as he shares specific steps you can take to prevent this terrible disease.

GET A COPY OF THESE BOOKS TODAY AT
www.drraystrand.com

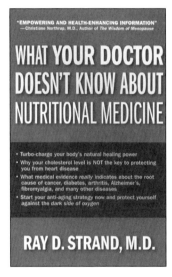

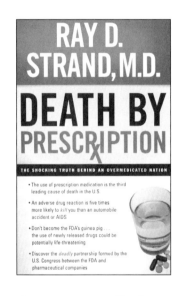

Dr. Strand's illumination of the body's silent enemy —oxidative stress — will astound you. But, more importantly, his research will equip you to protect or reclaim your nutritional health, possibly reversing disease and preventing illness.

Learn to protect yourself and your loved ones from the third leading cause of death in the US--legal medication. Dr. Strand exposes the dangers of an overmedicated society and the inherent risk of all prescription medication. He describes the "deadly partnership" that has developed between the pharmaceutical companies and the FDA.